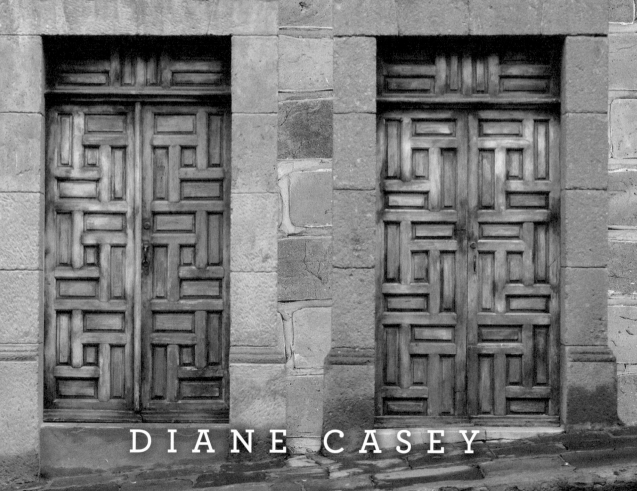

GREEN WALLS
AND
BROWN DOORS

DIANE CASEY

iUniverse books may be ordered through booksellers or by contacting:

iUniverse
1663 Liberty Drive
Bloomington, IN 47403
www.iuniverse.com
844-349-9409

ISBN: 978-1-6632-0507-0 (sc)
ISBN: 978-1-6632-0508-7 (e)

Library of Congress Control Number: 2020913166

Print information available on the last page.

iUniverse rev. date: 12/03/2021

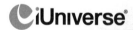

GREEN WALLS AND BROWN DOORS

Diane Casey

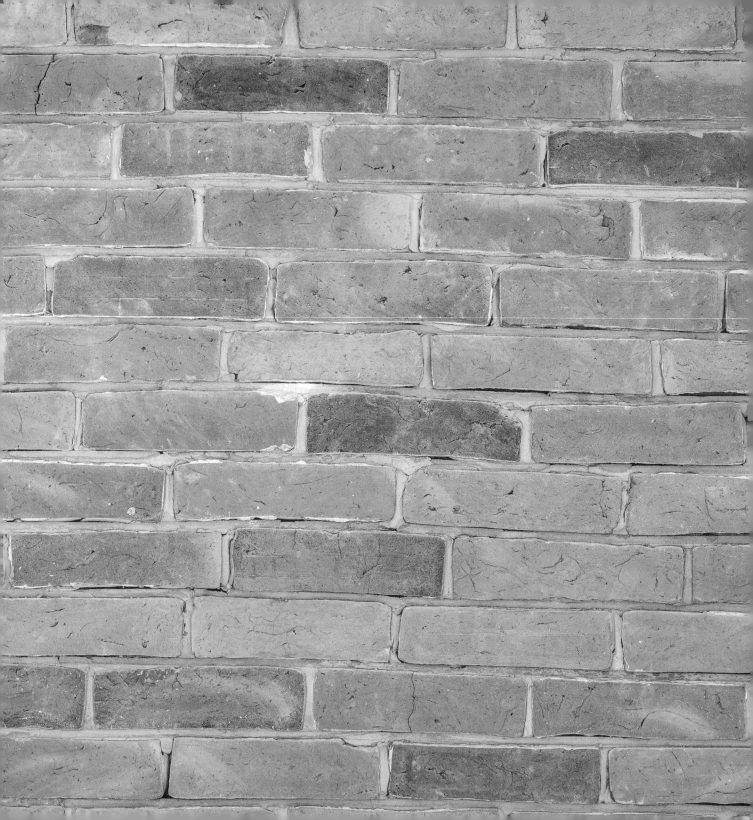

TABLE OF CONTENTS

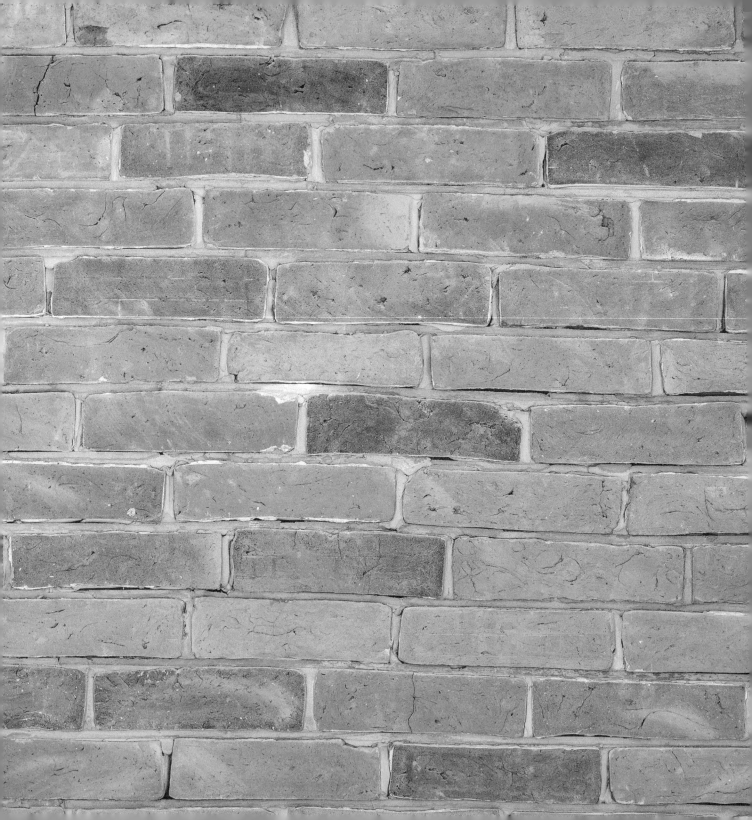

This work is based upon actual events, dialogue, and characters.

FORWARD

This book is dedicated to survivors and overcomers of Bipolar Disorder who fight to manage their mental health symptoms and admissions to mental health facilities. The undesirable falls, getting back up and never giving up hope, and desire to see what is around the next corner. I am also an overcomer of Bipolar Disorder that tore my family apart, and had ruled my life for many years. Eventuality I learned there are many shades of grey. Learning to be comfortable with the grey areas begins new healing in lives. Join me in reading my book; I will enjoy your company. It may help you or a loved one. Never give up hope.

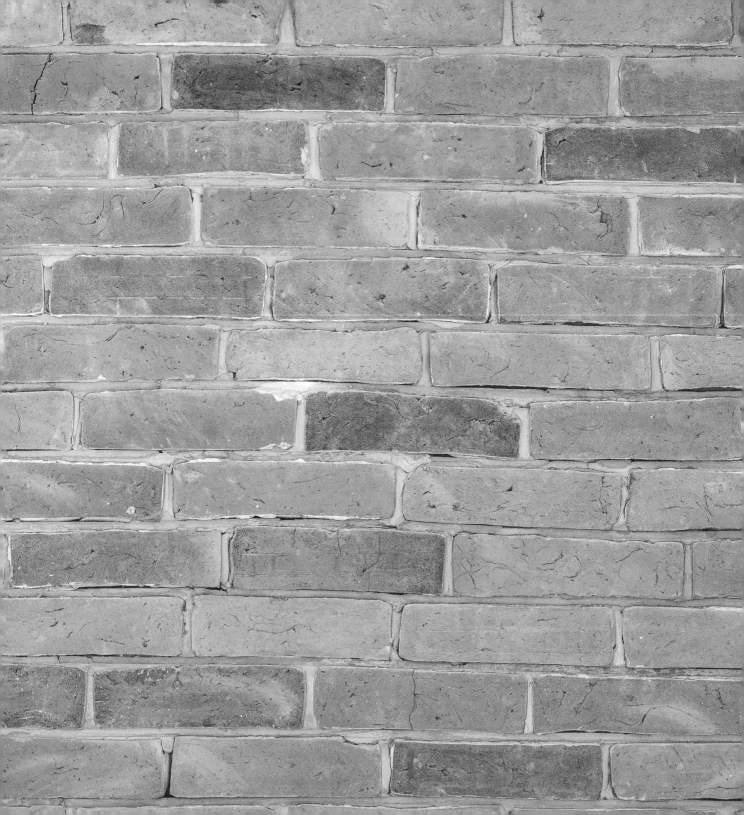

Chapter 1. In the beginning

Through the years, medications never helped; I was misdiagnosed. As Psychology advanced, it explained the behavior that fit me after the myriad of diagnoses. My diagnosis is BiPolar Disorder.

Families, in most cases, have the emotional tools to help their children through milestones of growth. Others do not have dynamic tools.

Age seven was a milestone in my life fraught with awful experiences. I wanted so much to be accepted, and when the teenage boys asked me to come into their tent, I was elated. At age seven, the neighborhood boys sexually abused me. In the tent, they pushed me down on the cot and stuck little sticks into me. I couldn't tell my parents as they would blame me. At the same time, I started to self-harm. I would dig my arms with a broken plastic ruler. My parents didn't know this because I wore long sleeves. I had no voice. The only way to deal with the pain and embarrassment was to swallow my shame.

At the same time, I started to self-harm. I would dig my arms with a broken plastic ruler. My parents didn't know this because I wore long sleeves. I had no voice. The only way to deal with the pain and embarrassment was to swallow my shame. Over time, I realized as parents remained wounded early in life, they tend to allow their hurt to trickle down to their children. It is not intentional; most parents do not mean to hurt their children.

I lacked the social skills to ask for what I needed. As I grew older, I knew I had the power to find the opportunity to discover new strengths and a new way of thinking. The purpose of this book is to reach down to your soul and let you know there is hope and in totality and growth. Some may think to take my words and ponder the meaning, and some may dismiss my words entirely. I seek to reach out to others who cry for some relief, have been hospitalized, and never validated.

Moving ahead a few years, I was eight, and the ministers' daughter was eight. We became fast friends. Debbie was the glue that held my life together and, both her parents were in the Salvation Army as ministers. They would transfer them every two to six years. Debbie and I shared stories about our lives, families, and hope. Debbie gave me new insights into her family life that was different from mine. She gave me hope. She gave me the hope there was something out there if I could hold on till age 18, I could find the right man and make a healthy family as Debbies parents had. Later I learned Debbie's Father was in a car accident that shattered the bones in his legs. Debbie's Father spent one year in Physical Therapy. When he was well enough, the family transferred to New York. It was time for Debbie to say goodbye I wrote to her once, and she responded, then I never heard from her again.; it was tough to let her go. When I entered Grammer school, I made new friends and enjoyed learning.

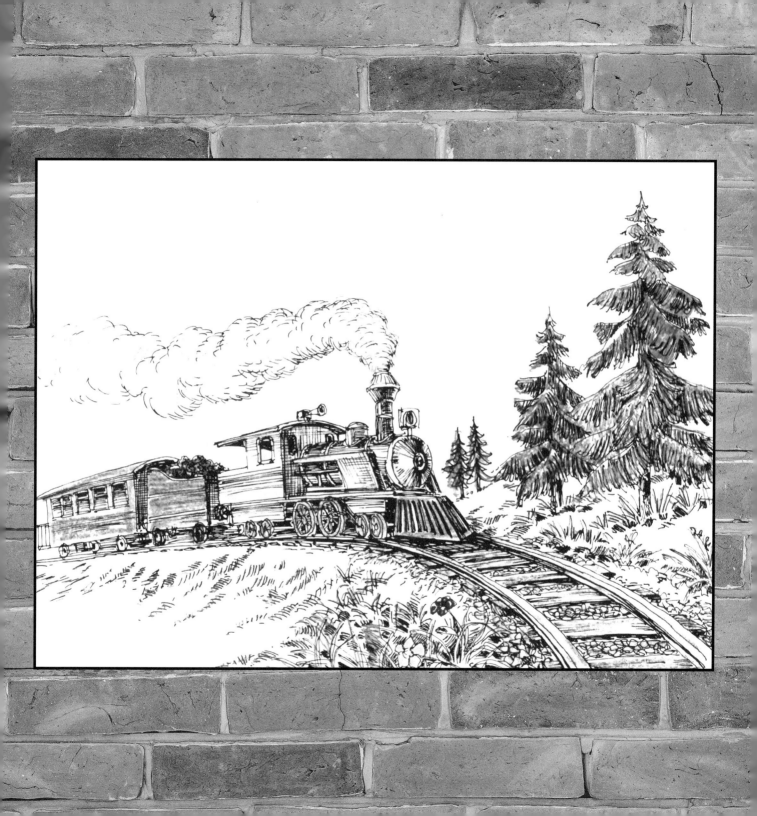

Chapter 2 . What is normal?

During my childhood years, I spent many an hour playing marbles, Cat women, and jacks. At the age of 12, things turned ugly, and I was bullied every day in school.

I saw my Father dull his pain in alcohol, so I would dull my pain by taking a whole bottle of pills. While waiting for the school bus, I confided in another student what I had done, and she reported it to the school staff.

When I transitioned from childhood to adolescence, I was deficient in many ways. I could no longer live with the trials of living in my home. I was admitted to a local hospital then transferred to the State Hospital. The nightmare began, and I had little knowledge of what I had to grow through to become the person I am today. My first impression of the building was how big it was. Walking in, I saw a few offices. I said goodbye to my Mom, relieved I was no longer had to live in fear and went on to what I thought was security. Lucia, the head attendant, met us at the door and put on a vastly different face for my Mom. The Dining room was the first room we walked through. It was barren and painted solid yellow.

I wondered how people could eat in a sad-looking such as this. As we continued walking, we came to a locked door, and Lucia took out her key chain and unlocked the door. That is when I first saw the Green Walls and Brown doors. The Green Walls and Brown Doors would haunt me for many years and the secrets they held. But for now, being new, I was scrutinized by the other girls. I was quiet but mindful of my surroundings. During the time I was there, I was in a group of 5 girls. I was so afraid I could not let myself swallow. If I swallowed, it would make a noise and draw attention to me. All I did was stare out the window and not move a muscle.

Over the next few months, as I settled in, the rage I built up over the years began to seep out of me. I was continually rebellious, angry, and violent. Lucia was the one who physically restrained me due to my wild mood swings and many a time tied me down to the bed and left me for hours. Lucia tied me to the bed one time as she was closing the seclusion room door. I told her I bit my thumb, and she said is it bleeding? I said yes, and she said good and locked the door behind her. Another time Lucia taunted me in the dining room to the point I hit her on the back. Lucia turned around, grabbed my arm, and twisted my arm so far up my back; I thought she would dislocate my shoulder. Daily, swept away with anger, was a surge I could not control. Like my Dad, I would break windows using my fist and cut my arms with the glass. I would bang my head on the wall until the room spun around. The hospital staff decided to send me to the most violent ward of adult women. One day they put me in seclusion with leather straps and fastened me to the bed. After they left, I heard no one. They put me far away so no one could listen to me, My right foot began to hurt, and I looked down and saw my right foot had turned blue.

I started screaming for help before realizing it was just Jesus and me in a tender companionship. I had no one else to help me if I had lost my foot, and no one could ever take that moment of Jesus and me away from me. Fortunately, someone came in and saw my blue foot and quickly released me.

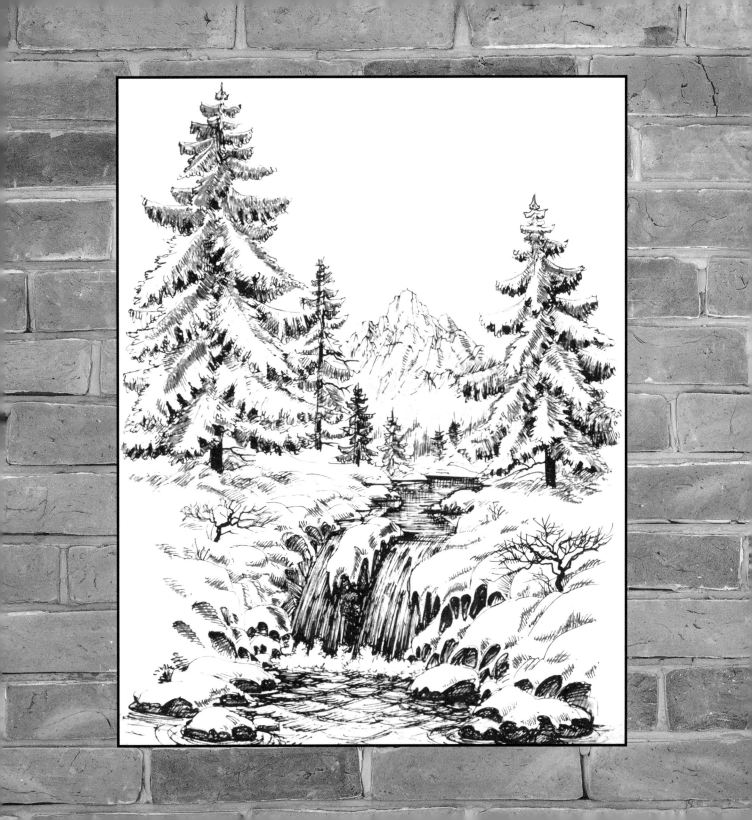

Chapter 3. On the outside, looking in.

To continue, some parents don't know what it's like being locked up and always restrained to a bed while hospital staff says I am okay. Many don't have a clue. I entered the State Hospital with the Green Walls and Brown doors from age 12 to 17; I stared at those walls and the secrets they held.

I never stopped to think of the family I left behind. I thought I'd be entering a world of security, but the opposite happened. Countless times you would find me tied to the bed for hours on end. With no knowledge to relieve the torment. I found ways of coping. The register system in my room is connected to the next room and is set up for heat and talking to one another; no matter how mentally challenged, we comforted each other.

Instead of the Hospital, my care moved into the hands of relatives. They sent me to a cult down south; they did horrible things to me in the name of Jesus. The cold tub of water, cold showers, paddlings, hogtied. As soon as I could, I left there, and my life began to turn for the better. I never spent a day in a High School classroom but went on to get my GED and two college degrees.

One day a staff approached me and said I needed to take a bath h; the Doctors wanted to talk to me, and I needed to be ready for them. One thing about young people in Woodstock is that I always wear jeans and an Indian-style shirt. That is the normalcy of a teenager at that time. In the Tub room. they took away my clothes and replaced them with a Ward dress and bobby socks.; I looked like the typical mental health patient. I waited in a large room called the day room. I heard the doctors approach the room, but they never came in to speak to me. They murmured amongst themselves then they were gone. No one came to talk to me; they came in to observe me. I was shocked and disappointed.

The outcome of the Doctor's observation? At the time, the hospital used shock treatment without the medications they have today. They also did lobotomies as a last resort. They called my parents for a meeting and said the only hope for me was a lobotomy. My parents said, no, If my parents said yes, I would have lost my soul.."

Eventually, due to the medication they put me on, I was in control enough to transfer back to the adolescent ward. I was labeled chronic and needing long-term care. To pass the time away, I listened to my music to settle my emotions. Lucia was still a force to be reckoned with; I learned to avoid her at all costs. I did not like her, and she was a constant threat to me. Then there were the dear souls on the staff who understood me. They were such a comfort to me. They used validation that is a powerful tool. Validation will pick you when you can't get up by yourself. When other people tell you what a great person you are and what a great job you're doing, that plants a seed to validate yourself. In the meantime, my Mom and sisters remained involved in my life, and they would come and see me every weekend we went to sit on the grass next to the duck pond we had on campus. We threw some potato chips in the direction of the ducks. The next thing we knew, a line of ducks came quacking in our direction. We grabbed our chips and ran away as fast as we could. Other times we spent Saturday afternoons bowling. On the way back to the hospital, my Mom and I would stop at a country store and buy bag chips and a soft drink. That was what

I enjoyed it the most and would wait until I got back to the ward to eat my snack. I never really missed my parents and thought they would live a long time - enough time for me to eliminate the bitterness and hurt I felt. Before my Dad died from Congestive Heart Failure, he was sorry for all the pain he caused me. I thanked him for the apology, told him that I loved him, then did not know what to say after that.

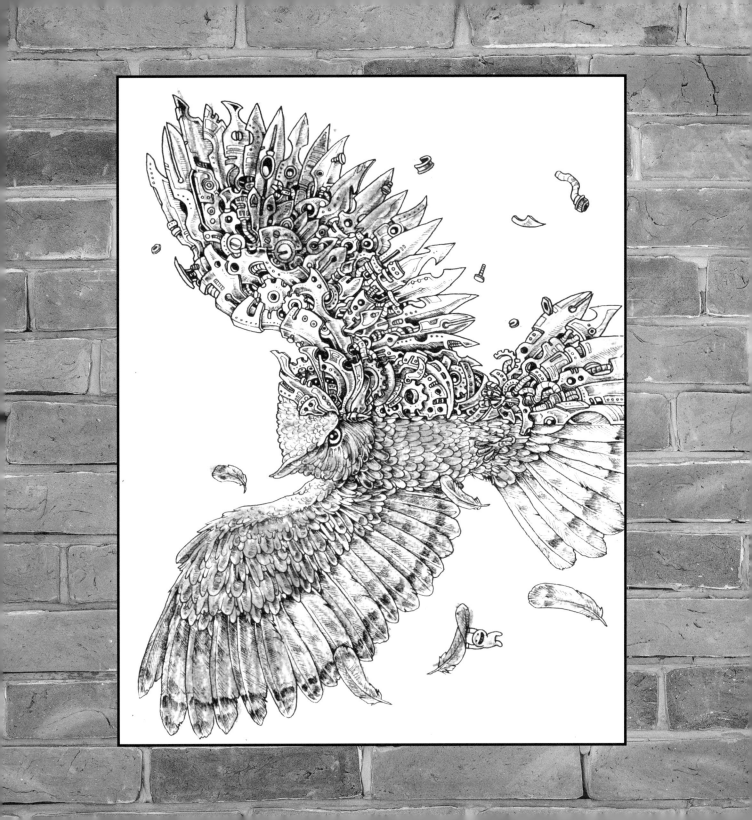

Chapter 4. Captive

At 17 and getting close to adulthood, the time was near to leave the Adolescent ward, and I was to return to and go back to the Adult ward. It was too much for me. I sobbed repeatedly, and a therapist I worked with said she could hear the fear I had when I cried. My Social Worker knew I had few options. My Mother contacted some very dear relatives to arrange to be put me in their care. The staff at the hospital agreed to turn me over to my relatives and take responsibility for my care.

Many years ago, when I was age 7, I told my Aunt I wanted to live in a place where they loved Jesus all the time. At the age of 17, my Aunt and Uncle found a place for me called "The Move," A group of Christians who believed the Lord was coming back soon. Furthermore, people should become empty vessels for the Lord to work through. It was the dawn of a new life for me. I will never forget but forgive.

I lived with my Aunt and Uncle for two weeks. They finalized my plans to move me to the Christian Group, the Church of God in Eupors, Mississippi. Before I left my Aunt's and Uncle's care, I poured all my medications down the sink as a move of faith., never thinking of the side effects stopping the medicine abruptly. I was on my way to the Church in a car with one of their members driving. By the time I arrived at the Church's door doorstep, I was in full-blown withdrawal. The Group leaders, John and Bambi, got me settled into their trailer. They immediately put me in one-on-one care of the younger leadership. The more they preached Jesus to me, the more I rebelled.

The only reason I could think I rebelled against the Jesus I loved was that I was angry with the way they dealt with those who rebelled. They hogtied me on the floor until my thighs burned. I was tied to a chair and made to wear headphones listening to Gospel songs for hours. They put me in the cold shower. They filled the bathtub With cold water and ice and held me under until I calmed down. When I started screaming, they would cover my mouth and nose so I could not breathe. They tied a rope around my waist, and I had to run in circles in the mud until I was too tired to fight. There were paddlings with a belt, a switch, or wooden paddles. The casting out of demons would take hours until the Elders thought the beast was gone. They focused on demons as they did on Jesus. I got to the point I believed there were demons everywhere, and they would get me if I left John and Bambi. If you did not respond to the love of Jesus, you were giving in to the flesh. In direct opposition, we had good times too. The praise services around the campfire. Sitting on the front porch, listening to the whippoorwills, someone softly playing, singing a Gospel song in the background. Those were the times I held on to, the most peaceful times of my life.

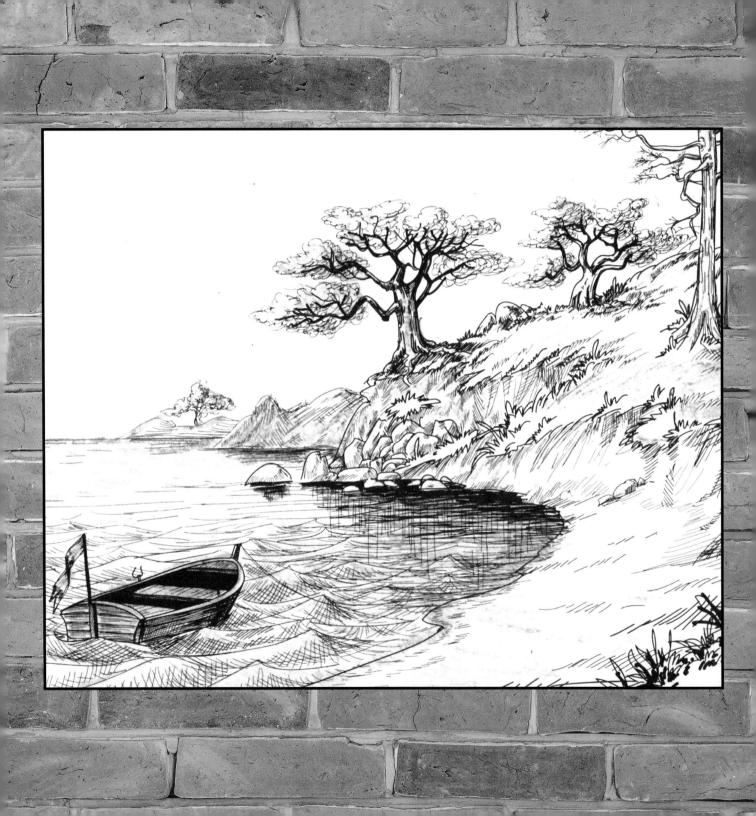

Chapter 5. Confused

Through the horrendous experiences done to me, I strangely grew to love John and Bambi. They never left my side; I identified with their mission so that I could survive. I can't entirely agree with the methods they used and never will, but I felt their heart was in the right place. The Church of God was also called the farm. The farm was growing, and one new member noticed the treatment I received. This new member escaped from the farm and went to the sheriff's office to report he saw. Soon, the sheriffs were at the farm, and the Attorney General got involved. The Attorney General's made the decision I would have counseling sessions with a psychologist once a week. After a while of meeting, I told the psychologist about the cold water treatments. John immediately denied such a treatment ever occurred. The following week I had a scuffle on the floor with John and Bambi, and I dislocated my knee and could not walk very well. The psychologist came out to see me and wanted me to walk with him to the other side of the farm; I told him I could not. I found out later they had a car waiting for me and planned on taking me away so they could De-program me; that ride never happened.

At age 21, John and Bambi decided it was time to leave and drove me from Mississippi to my parents' home in New Hampshire, where I again was admitted to the State Hospital.

The hospital was not the same as I remember. Methods had changed; all was pro-active and for the better. I never spent a day in a high school classroom or graduated from the eighth grade. I now had the opportunity to get my GED, and I did. It was not an easy road since I missed so much. Slowly but surely, I kept up and graduated, complete with cap and gown. I was overwhelmed with my accomplishment; I cried with joy. It did not end there; the hospital discharged me to a group home. Unfortunately, the Woman who owned the house was interested in the money; It was not a nurturing environment. I give her credit; she did try, but she did not have what it took to run a group home.

I slowly began to realize I lacked the social skills to ask for what I needed. As I grew older, I knew I had the power to find the opportunity to discover new strengths and a new way of thinking. The purpose of this book is to reach down to your soul and let you know there is hope and in totality and growth. Some may think to take my words and ponder the meaning, and some may dismiss my words entirely. I seek to reach out to others who cry for some relief, have been hospitalized, and never validated. What is my life like having BiPolar?

Picture yourself outside at night, no coat. The weather is below zero, and you have no building to protect yourself in, so cold and nowhere to go. How are you going to live? How will you survive? That's, to me, the depressive state of BiPolar. The hyper side of Bipolar is a thirst from the fire around you and in you. You can try to stop it, but the torturing flames are at your heels. It would be best to move to get out of the heat, but the fire won't let you. Is there a way to get out of the hell of both sides? Medications? Perhaps I've taken a myriad of medicines until the Doctor found one that changed my life completely. I finally learned to feel normal (at least to me). I have learned to laugh at myself. How to find strength amid a battle so intense I thought I would wither up and die.

One story that stands out in my mind is after my husband died at age 50 and my son was 14. My son started getting in trouble with the law. I had to sell my house and find the courage to take my son to a place of support. I took him to a facility in Florida that would give him help, and I went with him. My son flourished there; I did not. At 18, my son left and joined the Air Force. He never returned. He left the facility and never wrote to me, never called. Every day I prayed for him, sent him Holiday messages, etc. Every day I had to have faith in his return, and finally, my dedication paid off. My son sent me a message on social media on mothers Day. If God has faith in us, then we have to have in him.

Chapter 6. Stormy Weather

My Father had a rough life. He grew up in an Irish Catholic family where beer was the standard to dull physical and emotional pain. My Dad learned from his Dad how to deal with emotions. His Mother passed away when my Dad was only 16; he told me how abandoned he felt years later. He talked about his twin sisters, who passed away as infants. It was during the time of the Spanish flu. Dad never talked much about his family. I know he lived in a big house with a family that traveled from Ireland till they were on their feet. Many changed their last names, and many family members came over to join loved ones before them. Dad was a good man, and I believe My Dad was Bipolar. For example, one minute, he was on a high then dropped to depths of despair. In the era I was born, new mothers remained in the hospital for a week.

Meanwhile, my Dad was trying to get a crib for me on credit; he wrote a cheerful letter to my Mom and delivered it to the hospital, and the nurses would pass out the mail.

The next day he reported he could not get a crib for me on credit and was despondent. The two set me up in a dresser drawer; they worked together to solve the problem. Those were the times we had fun with him when he was sober.

My Mom had a rough childhood also. {My sister Glenda's experience about our Mom.) My Grandfather had lost his wife in childbirth, leaving him with four little girls to raise. In the meantime, his sister-in-law had lost her husband, leaving her with four boys. They solved their dilemma by joining forces and combining their families. She cared for the children and the house while he worked and paid the bills. It was a wild and hectic, stressful existence, with the children falling through the cracks in the meantime. She strongly favored her boys over his girls, to the point where she would hit the girls to show the boys what they would get if they didn't get their way, life was tough for my Mother, and she couldn't wait to leave.

My Mom grew up in Northfield, Vermont. Norwich University is the center of the town, and when my Mom was a teenager, rumors circulated about her because it seemed she was always pregnant. With her reputation at stake, she chose to leave her hometown.

My Mom had 11 children, and only five of us survived. When she wanted to move to New Hampshire, her Father gave an ultimatum. Mom being so young with three children were forced to choose to bring two of her children with her or not go at all. She decided to move to New Hampshire, taking with her two little daughters. Thus, I (Glenda, my sister) ended up shuffled from place to place. When she arrived in New Hampshire, she went to live with her Aunt Grace. My Mom lost the address and had little knowledge of exactly where her Aunt lived. The cab driver drove around the neighborhood until she said, "that's it," as she recognized the apartment building number; she and my two sisters settled in. With Aunt Grace watching my two sisters, Mom had more time to herself.

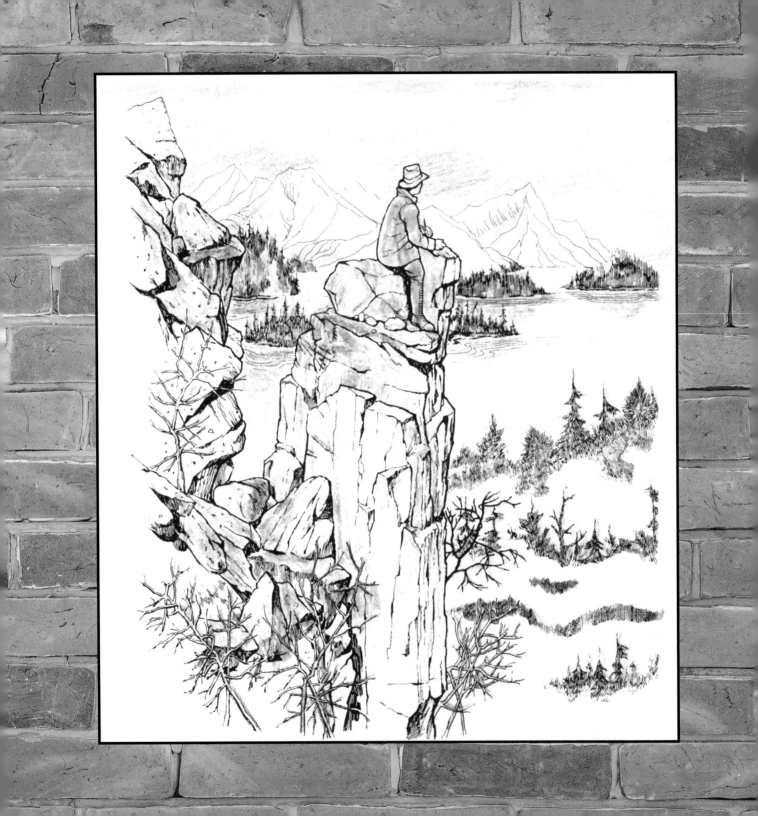

Chapter 7. Toxic abuse on the horizon.

Mom enjoyed meeting new people and socializing. My Mom and Dad met each other in a beer joint of all places, a recipe for disaster. They grew to love each other, and I was born out of wedlock. The honorable thing to do in that day was to marry the Woman so the child would have two parents in the household; they had to change the name on my birth certificate.

My Mother had a hard life at the height of the depression. When food ran low in our present household, my Mom made an adventure out of bread, butter, and sugar, sometimes mayo sandwiches when food was scarce in our home. Because of her experience during the depression, she became creative in cooking meals. My Mother did not have the social skills needed to raise a family, but I knew I loved her, and she loved me. Mom was a heavy smoker, as was my Dad. One day a preacher came to town. Clinton White. I still remember his name like it was yesterday. He was a charismatic Evangelist, and my Mom felt it was time to quit smoking. Reverend White prayed over her. My Mom stopped smoking. She came home giving the reverend credit and the love of her Jesus to see her through.

On the other hand, my Father accused Mom of sleeping with the reverend and that she would sleep with anyone. I can understand his barb against my Mom, after having 11 children with different fathers, but she never smoked again. I soon learned that my Dad was himself in the morning, and by the evening, he would be a different person. As soon as he got home from work, he would start drinking. Christmas morning was exciting and magical for me. Once, my Father stayed up all night to put together a pink bicycle for me. The color was perfect, and oh how I wanted to ride it, but in New Hampshire, we were sure of at least four more months of snow on the ground. Soon, our family had to deal with a sad situation looming in our lives.

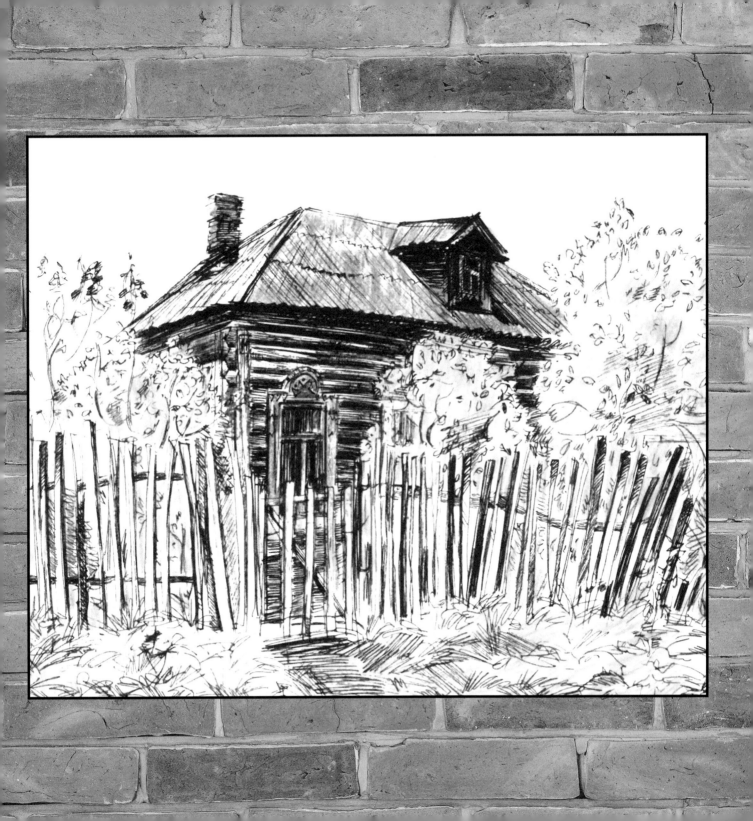

Chapter 8. A Great Loss

Let me introduce you to my sister Barbara. Barbara went through a lot in her life. She had many relationships over time but had one boyfriend she would ask him to buy a pack of cigarettes for her. Three days later, he would come back with the cigarettes; that was his pattern to disappear for days, but Barbara always took him back. I think Barbara looked for the love she never really received and was used to being abused. For all her trials, she always made you laugh; she turned the negative into a positive. Barbara became pregnant with her son Adam. When Adam was about 5 or 6, Barabra, Adam, and I walked past a convenience store. Adam wanted a candy bar; Barbara and I had no money. We could not buy him a candy bar, which has always haunted me. Then out of nowhere, it seemed Barbara it hard to breathe; finally, the Doctor had her wear oxygen all the time. Barbara and her son Adam moved into a house with Al (her boyfriend). One time, Barbara's screaming woke up Al. Her oxygen caught on fire when she went to light a cigarette. Al put out the fire with his hands. Barbara had a few scars on her face. Another time she was in the hospital she was unresponsive, and I went in every day and read to her. Every time I read something funny, her blood pressure would rise; she was hearing me. She had been in the hospital countless times. Then the day came; she told us she was tired and ready to let go. Surrounded by her family, she went to sleep and quietly passed on. I miss her.

I want to introduce my sister Marilyn. At age five, I witnessed What I believed to be the end of our family honor as I knew it. Marilyn was always the scapegoat. I think the reason for this is she rebelled against the toxic environment at home. She also had a reputation with the boys. I was in our pantry, off of the kitchen; my drunk Father stood in the middle of the kitchen and said to Marilyn, "I bet you would even make out with your stepfather" then he kissed her on her mouth and pushed on her breast. How horrible of him to cross the boundary of our family's integration.

My world cracked into shards of disbelief. I learned that I could not trust my parents in this development stage, and I was reluctant to trust others. My sisters and I have been through a lot; my family had a strange way of ignoring the elephant in the room. To this day, I have a hard time explaining it and understanding it. It was with my Mom that we connected. We had a bond when we needed to bond together. When we no longer needed the bonding, we quietly slipped away to the corners of our reality until the bonding was needed again. My sisters Marilyn and Barbara were good to me. They would take me places with their boyfriends.

One time (and I didn't know better), I lined up my sister's cigarettes end to end like a train out to the kitchen and around my Dad's chair. When he realized what I was doing, and the cigarettes belonged to my sisters, he made my sisters smoke a cigar. They were sick from the cigar and mad at me; I was only making train tracks. I've introduced each family member but have not touched on the whole family as a unit. I still remember the time my Father and Mother fought (again). My Father yelled at me to get my Mother out of the closet. She had run to the closet and closed the door. My Mom was yelling; I'm going to kill myself with this butcher knife. My Father yelled, "I'm going to put my hand in the flame of the gas stove." I stood frozen to the floor; I didn't know what to do; I was only four years old. Finally, I convinced my Mom to come out. How often did I have to run after my Mother barefoot in the snow, begging her to come home? She told me through her tears that she would come back for us. We feared being abandoned and left with our Father. My Mom returned home the same evening. The rough nights when the escalation at home forced my Mom to get us out of the house, and we stayed in hotels (and not the safest ones). At one hotel, a man came banging on the door asking for Charlie. I thought he would break down the door. Mom told us to be quiet, and I held my breath. Eventually, he went away. The next day, my Mom called Dad to see if he had calmed down. My Father begged us to come home, and he had bought lobsters. Lobsters were expensive, and we could not afford them. We returned home but still had to deal with the broken promises, and the violence continued.

One burst of anger from my Father happened, and he choked my Mom to the point of unconsciousness. My sister Barabra took a beer bottle and smashed it over our Father's head to stop him from strangling my Mom.

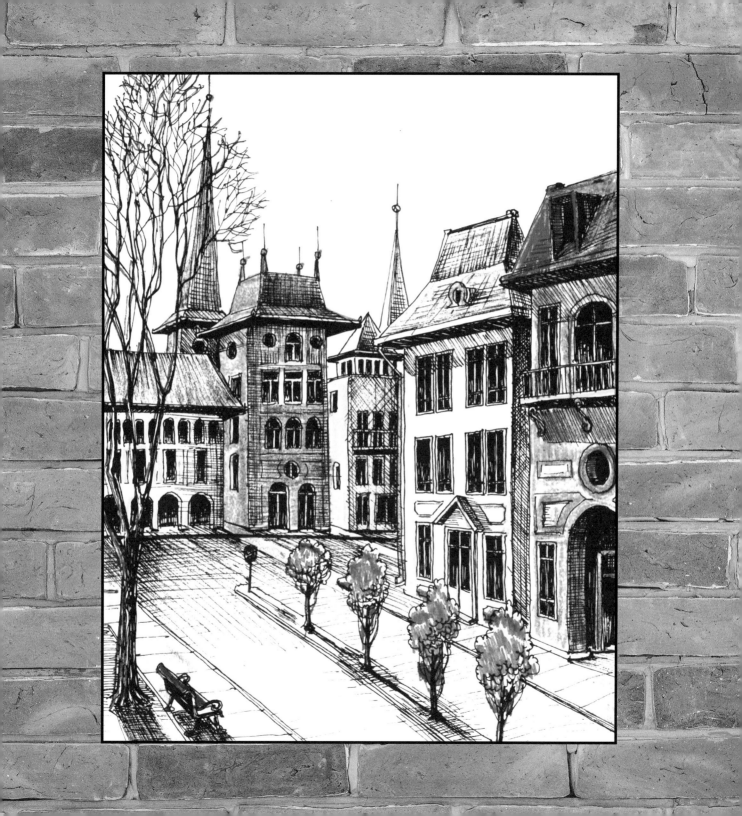

Chapter 9. Bad to better.

At age seven, I was sexually abused by the neighborhood boys. I was so happy when the teenage boys invited me into their tent. I felt so special to gain their attention. Once inside, they pushed me down on a cot they had and began inserting sticks in me. I can't go further with this as I have yet to heal completely. I started to self-harm. I would take plastic rulers and break them apart so I would have sharp edges. I would take the sharp edges and dig up my arms. The weather was cool, so I wore long sleeves, and no one noticed.

It took me years to realize our symptoms will, at times, rear their ugly head out of the blue. Out of the blue brings beautiful things to help us grow.

Be cautious of labels. It is easy to let labels define who you are. There are labels you have placed on yourself or others have placed on you. Bipolar is not who I am; I am uniquely Diane. It's easy to fall into the trap of a Bipolar diagnosis (or any diagnosis) that could define a bond with being who you are and bind your growth potential. I strongly suggest a need for change; be yourself and not a diagnosis. Doing so is to win the battle within us. I realized I had hope. My definition of hope is determination, spirituality, and courage.

However, I had difficulties holding a job. One job, in particular, changed my life completely. I walked into a Shell gas station. Behind the counter was an employee that when I saw him, my heart fluttered. I met the man that would be my future husband, and we were so in love. Tim told me when I left the station. He took out my application to see if I was single.

A couple of years into our relationship, we had a baby boy named Joshua. At age 2, I would read a book about clouds to him. To my amazement, he memorized each page of that book. He knew how to tell time at age 4. The mystery about Joshua was why he did not make eye contact or could not understand social cues. We took him to the Doctor (neurologist), and she diagnosed Joshua on the autism spectrum. One day, Joshua told me his medicine made him feel awful. I called his Doctor and told her what was going on. The Doctor said for Joshua to go one week without the meds.

Within that week, Joshua began to make eye contact and recognizing social cues. One day a student in his class bumped into a table, knocking everything to the floor. The student (she) tried to pick everything up. Joshua got up from his seat, knelt beside her, and started picking things up with her. The classroom that laughed at her got up from their chairs and started picking items up. Joshua always had a tender heart and is/was very intelligent. I soon learned I had an older sister named Glenda. When I met her, the first thing I did was climb onto her lap with my book of fairy tales. In she read it to me. One day, Glenda came to visit us when Joshua was 2. He climbed up into Glendas lap with his cloud book and asked her to read it to him. Then we went out onto the driveway and saw a dandelion pushing its way through solid rock. That was amazing to see.

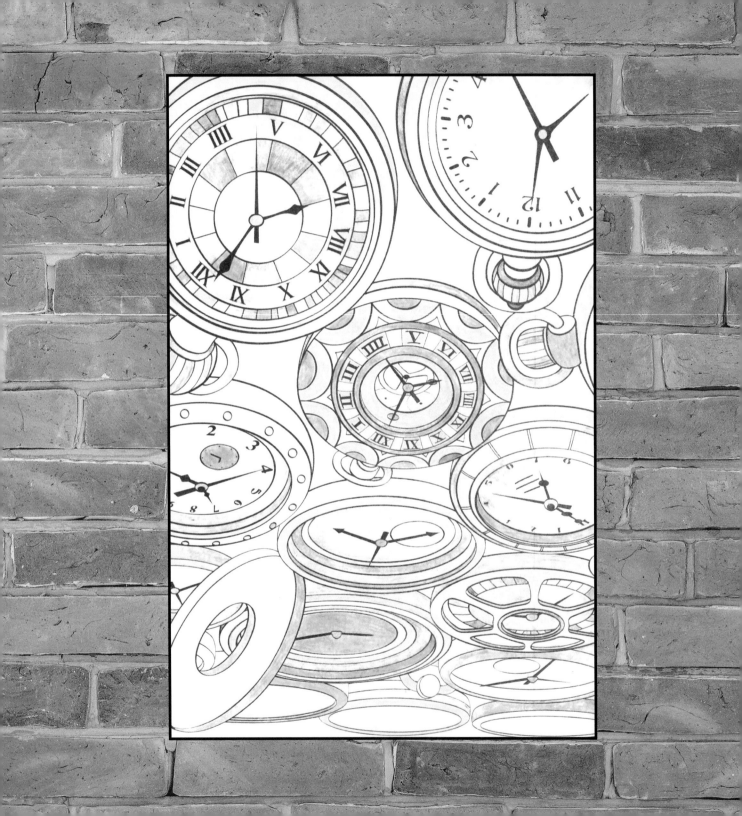

Chapter 10. I lost my true love.

Backing up a little bit, Tim and I ended up getting well-paying jobs. Tim worked as a cable operator, and I worked as an Executive Director for a non-profit agency for people with mental illness. Both Tim and I worked at our jobs for 15 years before his death. When we bought our house, it was a dream come true. Tim and I had precious times until Tim died; Tim was only 50 when he passed. He died from a massive heart attack. In the ER, the Doctor working on Tim asked me if I wanted to continue the life-saving procedure. I looked at Tim's face, and he looked so tired, like he had been through a war. I couldn't let him suffer any longer, and I said no, don't go on. My Tim had passed. Joshua (at the age of 14) was home at the time and, of course, shaken by watching his Father die in my arms.

After Tim died, I felt like I had lost my rudder and could no longer steer the boat. When Tim passed away, I lost my anchor. Joshua, who was 14 at the time, watched Tim die, and we could not save him.. After Tim's burial, our home life became a toxic environment. All I could do was get Joshua up for school, make sure he had food to eat, and wash his clothes. Other than that, all I could do was sleep all day on the couch. Our little dog stayed at the foot of the sofa near me, and he knew I was upset.

I couldn't think of how to clean my house; our Christmas tree was still up, and it was May. To this day, I can't remember the date he died. Joshua started to get into trouble with the law. I almost lost Joshua to Child Services. Joshua needed family support. I made sure Joshua was fed and washed his clothes got him up for school. Other than that, I fell asleep on the couch all day with our American Eskimo at my feet. Joshua was getting into trouble with the law for vandalizing cars. He got off with a warning, but I feared that Joshua's behavior would get worse. Joshua and I needed structure in our lives; we were like leaves blowing in the wind. The alternative I had was to move to Florida, back with John and Bambi. Their philosophy had changed. John and Bambi replaced the methods of cruelty and no longer used the punishments as they did before. As Joshua flourished and adjusted well to his new surroundings, I did not. I became more depressed every day. My emotions ruled my behavior, and I could help but dig myself deeper into my depression. The Church had to Baker Act me.

I was committed to a psych hospital against my will for 72 hours. I knew I could never return to John and Bambi. They said Joshua could stay with them, and it was best to leave him in their care. At age 17, he joined the Air Force. I transferred from one assistant Living Facility to another ALF to another due to my behavior. Transferred from one Assistant Living Facility to another, I was looking for a home and would sabotage myself, so I had to leave. I realized my action would not end until I found a home. I found a nursing care facility that cared for physical issues and specialized in mental health behaviors. I finally found my home in Greenville, Florida.

The next subject in my book I need to include is my sister Glenda's view of my Mothers struggle with a massive stroke. This paragraph may seem out of place, but it is important to me. My sister Glenda put our family unity into perspective by summing up the following. G Glenda said she had her story to share about Mom's death. My friend Barb drove me from Vermont to New Hampshire. We spent the day at a gathering; Mom was there too. Everyone had left, and I knew Barb was anxious to get home. I went over and gently told Mom we were leaving. An anguished scream came from her lips. "Nooooo! Don't go" I waited a while and settled her down, then we quietly left. I cried for the two-hour trip home. Within minutes of my arrival at the house, the phone rang. My sister Carol told me they did not know if Mom would make it through the night. I instantly grabbed my keys and headed back to New Hampshire. It was a tearful and hasty journey back.

By the Grace of God, I made the trip with no injury to others or myself. I do not know how fast I drove; I do know I was passing car after car, praying fervently to get there before Mom was gone. Her room was full of people when I got there, including the pastor of her Church. I flew into the room, tossed my purse onto a table. My car keys skidded across the floor and under the radiator. Mom was no longer talking or opening her eyes, but we knew she was hearing. My son and his wife had just learned the child they were expecting was a little girl. I told her that, and a joyous squeal came from her mouth. That was all. But I knew she had heard, and the news had given her a moment of joy.

There was a room adjacent to hers which family members could spend the night. A roll-out couch and maybe some recliners? I scarcely recall that night, but I do remember the feeling of family closeness and love.

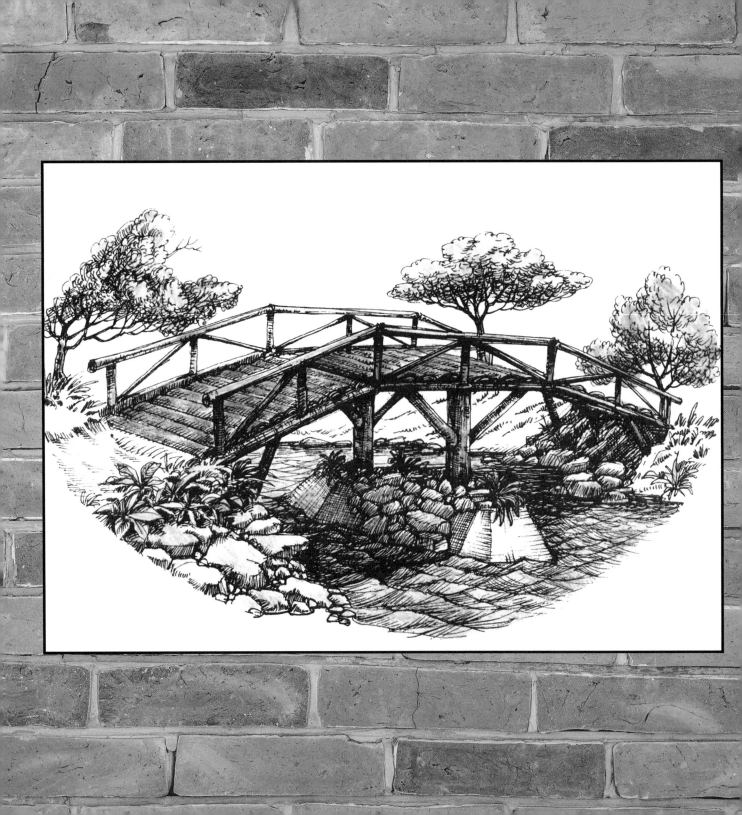

Chapter 11. Not again.

When I moved to Florida, I ended up at Florida State Hospital for four and a half years. I spent most of my time tied to a Gerry chair.

It had been several years since I heard from Joshua. He surprised me by contacting me on Mother's day in 2021. He is stationed in Florida, and I did not want to leave Florida if he wanted to see me and would not have so far to travel.

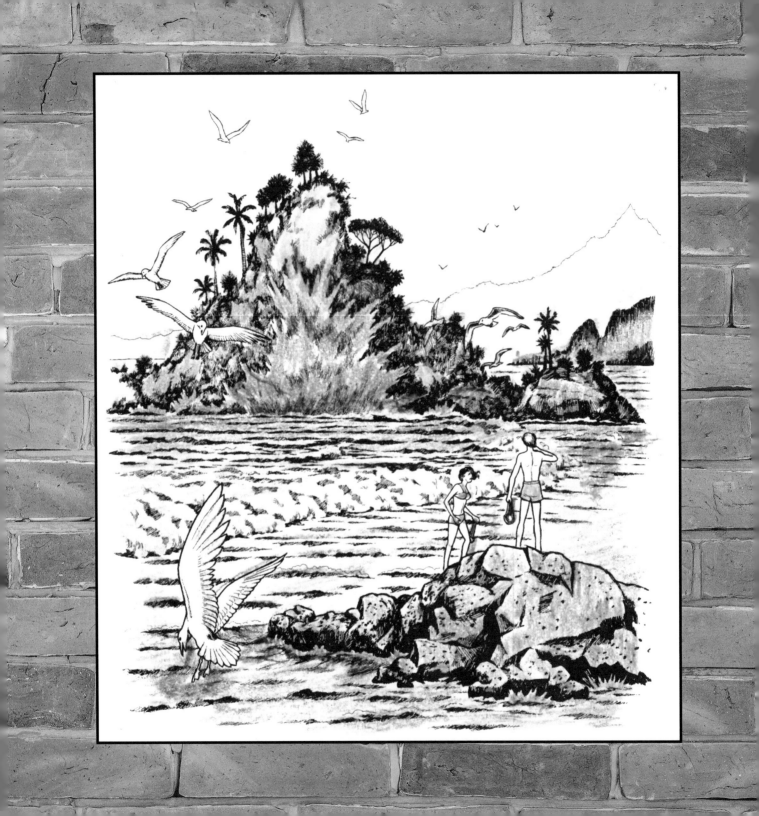

Chapter 12. Coming to an end.

I look back over the years and reflect on circumstances I could have handled differently. I cringe at some of the things I have done and said. I quietly grieve at what my life could have been if Tim lived. I have few regrets and cherish the many people who have crossed my path. I have learned to realize that each day, each moment is as precious as jewels. In January of 1999, I was diagnosed with Diastolic Congestive heart failure, and part of my lungs scarred from COPD. I also have kidney disease but have learned to manage my symptoms. I feel the time to share my story is now. I want my voice, my essence, heard. If it helps one person, then it is all worth it. Thank you for walking on my journey with me, and no matter what, do not give up hope.

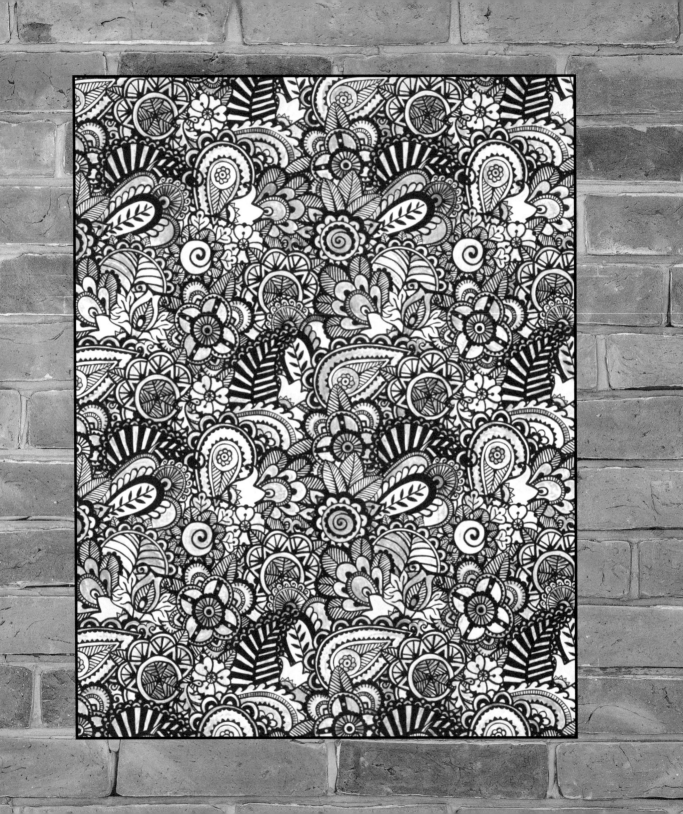

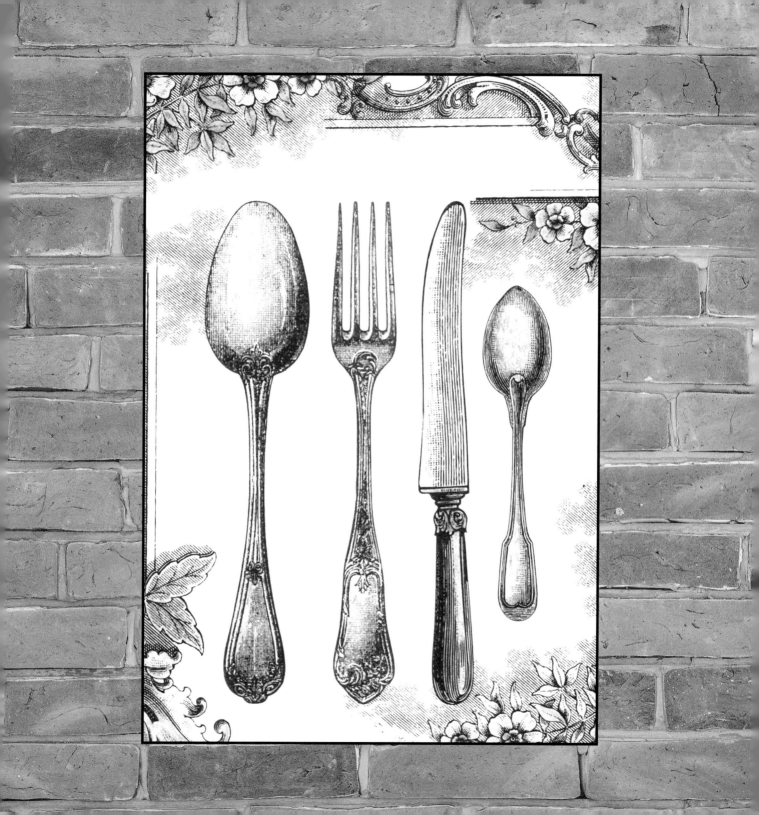

Printed in the United States
by Baker & Taylor Publisher Services